UNDERSTANDING

REFLEXOLOGY

FOR BEGINNERS

Discover Proven Methods For Enhancing Relaxation, Boosting Circulation, And Promoting Natural Healing Through Reflexology

DR. ALICIA SONYA

CONTENTS

DISCLAIMER

The information provided in this book is for educational and informational purposes only and is not intended as medical advice, diagnosis, or treatment. Always consult with a qualified healthcare professional before beginning any therapy, practice, or lifestyle change.

The author and publisher of this book make no representations or warranties regarding the accuracy, applicability, or completeness of the content presented. While every effort has been made to ensure the information provided is accurate and up-to-date, the field of health and wellness is constantly evolving, and the reader is advised to use discretion and seek professional guidance as needed.

This book contains references to individuals, products, websites, organizations, or other entities solely for informational purposes. The author and publisher do not endorse, sponsor, or affiliate with any of these references, nor do they receive any benefit from their inclusion. The mention of any names, trademarks, or products does not imply any association or endorsement.

The use of this book is solely at the reader's discretion. Neither the author nor the publisher shall be held liable for any damages, loss, or injury resulting from the use or misuse of the information contained herein.

ABOUT THIS BOOK

Understanding Reflexology For Beginners"
serves as an essential resource for individuals
eager to unlock the therapeutic power of
reflexology, offering a comprehensive, step-
by-step approach to understanding and
practicing this ancient healing art. At its core,
reflexology centers on stimulating specific
reflex points on the feet, hands, and ears to
promote overall health, reduce stress, and
relieve various types of discomfort. This guide
introduces readers to reflexology's
foundational concepts, explores its extensive
health benefits, and demonstrates how to
apply its techniques effectively. From the
historical roots of reflexology to the tools and
supplies required for practice, this guide helps

practitioners and enthusiasts alike appreciate the science and skill behind this art form, as well as its profound impact on wellness.

Understanding reflex points and zones is crucial for anyone practicing reflexology, as these areas on the body map directly to different organs and systems. This guide demystifies foot, hand, and ear reflex maps, illustrating the relationship between reflex points and specific ailments.

Readers will gain a solid grasp of energy zones, learn practical tips for locating reflex points accurately, and understand the value of consistency in practice to achieve the best results. Each section builds upon the previous one, equipping readers with the knowledge needed to identify reflex points and make reflexology a regular, beneficial part of their lives.

Mastering reflexology techniques is essential, and this guide thoroughly explains thumb and finger techniques, pressure application, and common errors to avoid. Warming up and relaxing techniques are included to ensure that every session is both safe and effective, making reflexology accessible to those just starting their practice. Safety tips help readers prevent strain or overexertion, fostering a more comfortable experience. Additionally, detailed instructions are provided for the foundational techniques that form the backbone of effective reflexology practice, supporting readers in their journey from beginners to confident practitioners.

Specialized sections on foot, hand, and ear reflexology offer readers targeted approaches for these different areas. Foot reflexology provides an accessible entry point, with detailed information on preparing the feet, locating key reflex points, and sequencing techniques for a smooth, therapeutic session. Self-reflexology techniques allow readers to reap these benefits at home.

For hand reflexology, this guide explores the unique advantages of working with the hands and includes techniques that can easily be integrated into daily routines. Ear reflexology, or auricular reflexology, offers quick relief for various issues and includes key reflex points and techniques for issues like headaches and stress.

Each section equips readers with specialized techniques, promoting a well-rounded and adaptable reflexology practice.

Reflexology's effectiveness in stress relief and relaxation is a highlight of this guide. Readers will discover how reflexology soothes the nervous system, reduces anxiety, and supports better sleep through calming reflex points. Practical advice on creating a tranquil environment for sessions is provided, ensuring readers maximize reflexology's relaxation benefits.

For those interested in pain management, this guide details reflex points and techniques specifically aimed at alleviating headaches, migraines, joint pain, digestive discomfort, and circulatory issues. With easy-to-follow steps, readers can use reflexology to manage pain holistically and enhance their overall sense of well-being.

Additionally, this guide addresses common concerns and questions, clarifying reflexology's safety for various individuals and explaining the key differences between reflexology and massage. Practical advice on how often to practice reflexology and when to avoid or limit sessions guides readers, helping them develop a sustainable routine.

For readers new to reflexology, a troubleshooting section tackles issues such as handling sensitive reflex points, addressing soreness, and improving technique.

Myths and misconceptions are debunked, helping readers develop a clear, informed understanding of reflexology's potential.

Whether one is just beginning or seeking to deepen their understanding, "Complete Guide to Reflexology" serves as a comprehensive, insightful companion, empowering readers to embrace reflexology as a transformative tool for health and well-being.

CHAPTER ONE

Introduction To Reflexology

Reflexology is a therapeutic practice based on the principle that specific points on the feet, hands, and ears correspond to different organs and systems in the body. By applying pressure to these areas, reflexology aims to promote relaxation, reduce pain, and improve overall health. This holistic therapy is widely used to relieve stress and tension, stimulate circulation, and support the body's natural healing processes. Reflexology sessions can be performed by trained professionals or through self-treatment techniques for a calming experience.

Reflexologists use maps to identify zones and points on the feet and hands that correlate with specific body systems. For example, the big toe represents the head and brain, while the arch of the foot corresponds to the spine. By stimulating these areas, reflexologists aim to influence the body's energy flow, known as "Qi" in traditional Chinese medicine, to restore balance and wellness.

Sessions usually begin with a warm-up, gently massaging the feet or hands to relax muscles and improve circulation. The therapist or individual then applies pressure on target points with their thumbs or fingers, holding and releasing each spot before moving to the next.

Each point is massaged in a sequence that aims to provide relief, release blockages, and promote holistic health.

What Is Reflexology?

Reflexology is a type of alternative therapy that targets pressure points in the feet, hands, and ears to promote healing throughout the body. It's based on the theory that the body's various systems and organs have specific reflex points in these areas, which can be stimulated to bring about health benefits. Through precise thumb and finger techniques, reflexologists activate these points, aiming to reduce tension, enhance circulation, and improve the body's natural healing mechanisms.

In a typical reflexology session, practitioners focus on specific zones of the feet or hands, targeting reflex points that align with particular organs or body systems.

By pressing these points, they aim to send a "signal" to the related area within the body, releasing tension and allowing energy to flow freely. Reflexology follows a structured map, but sessions can be tailored to the individual's needs, whether they are seeking stress relief, pain management, or increased vitality.

Understanding reflexology doesn't require extensive knowledge of anatomy, as the focus is on using maps of the feet and hands. Beginners can start with simple techniques by pressing on areas associated with stress or tension, such as the reflex points for the spine and head located along the inner edges of the feet and big toes. Reflexology offers a straightforward yet effective way to engage with holistic self-care at home.

Brief History Of Reflexology

The roots of reflexology trace back to ancient civilizations, with early forms of reflexology found in Egypt, China, and India. Historical records show that Egyptian wall paintings depicted similar foot massage practices around 2330 BC, while traditional Chinese medicine has long held the belief in "Qi" energy flowing through specific pathways. In China, reflexology practices were used to encourage this flow of energy, and the technique evolved as part of a holistic approach to health.

Modern reflexology began to take shape in the early 20th century, thanks to Dr. William Fitzgerald, who introduced "zone therapy" in the United States. Dr. Fitzgerald theorized that the body could be divided into ten vertical zones, each one running from the top of the head to the toes and fingers. This zonal concept later evolved into what we now recognize as reflexology, with specific pressure points mapped onto the feet, hands, and ears.

Further development was carried out by Eunice Ingham, a physiotherapist who created the first comprehensive foot reflexology chart in the 1930s. Her work laid the foundation for reflexology as we know it today, making it more accessible and applicable to health and wellness.

Today, reflexology is recognized and practiced globally, providing people with a natural and supportive way to enhance their well-being.

Key Benefits For Health And Wellness

Reflexology is widely celebrated for its ability to promote relaxation, reduce stress, and support general health. The gentle pressure applied to reflex points can alleviate muscle tension and encourage deep relaxation, which, in turn, lowers levels of cortisol, a hormone associated with stress. Many people turn to reflexology as a non-invasive way to unwind and bring balance to the mind and body.

A notable benefit of reflexology is its role in improving circulation. By stimulating specific points, reflexologists help increase blood flow to targeted organs and tissues, which can support healing and rejuvenation. Improved circulation is essential for transporting oxygen and nutrients throughout the body, helping organs to function optimally. Those with circulation issues or swelling may find reflexology particularly helpful as it naturally promotes fluid balance and movement.

Additionally, reflexology is often used for pain management. People suffering from chronic conditions like headaches, migraines, back pain, or arthritis report reduced discomfort and improved mobility after regular reflexology sessions.

The therapy is also believed to support the body's detoxification processes, helping to eliminate toxins and boost immune function, which can lead to improved health and energy levels.

How Reflexology Works On The Body

Reflexology works by focusing on reflex points located primarily on the feet, but also on the hands and ears. These points correspond to specific organs and body systems, allowing reflexologists to target areas indirectly through pressure. When a reflex point is stimulated, it is believed to send a signal through the nervous system to the associated organ, promoting relaxation and supporting the body's healing response.

Each foot is mapped with zones representing different parts of the body, from the head to the feet. Reflexologists begin by applying gentle but firm pressure to these zones, holding and pressing each point for a few seconds before moving to the next. For instance, pressing on the arch of the foot corresponds to the digestive system, potentially helping those with digestive issues. As practitioners work through the points, they use various techniques, such as walking their thumb over each area, to stimulate different systems.

Reflexology's effects are holistic, often enhancing the function of multiple body systems simultaneously. For example, working on the point for the adrenal gland may help alleviate stress, while pressure on the lymph nodes can support immune function. This method of indirect treatment makes reflexology unique, as it offers a non-invasive approach to health and wellness that focuses on balancing the whole body.

Basic Tools And Supplies You'll Need

Getting started with reflexology doesn't require many tools, but there are a few essentials that can enhance your experience. First, a comfortable chair with good back support is important, especially for at-home sessions. Reflexologists typically work with the feet elevated on a footrest or cushioned stool to provide easy access and encourage relaxation. Soft lighting and calming music can also help create a soothing environment for effective therapy.

A reflexology chart is crucial, especially for beginners, as it maps the specific reflex points and zones on the feet and hands. These charts help guide the session by showing exactly where to apply pressure to target particular areas of the body. Many people find reflexology tools like small massage sticks or rollers useful for applying firm, steady pressure, though they aren't necessary for starting.

Lastly, using an unscented massage lotion or oil can help hands glide smoothly over the skin, reducing friction and making the experience more comfortable. Avoid applying too much, as a firm grip is needed to press into the reflex points effectively.

With these simple tools, you can practice reflexology comfortably at home, supporting your journey towards a relaxed and balanced state of mind and body.

CHAPTER TWO

Understanding Reflex Points And Zones

Reflex points are specific spots on the feet, hands, and ears that correspond to different organs, glands, and body systems. Reflexologists believe that applying gentle pressure to these points can stimulate energy flow, reduce tension, and improve overall wellness.

The concept rests on the idea that the body's different areas are mapped out across reflex points, allowing targeted pressure to affect the entire system positively. Recognizing these points and zones can empower you to take charge of your health, especially when dealing with minor issues like headaches or fatigue.

Reflex zones are the vertical and horizontal sections that divide the body and are mirrored on the feet, hands, and ears.

Imagine these zones as invisible pathways or channels of energy that connect reflex points with corresponding organs. For example, the vertical zones align from head to toe, meaning a reflex point on the big toe could influence the head, while one on the heel could affect lower body regions. This systematic approach helps practitioners address specific body areas more effectively.

In practice, you'll identify reflex points by using diagrams that display foot, hand, and ear maps. Begin by gently palpating the area, applying light to moderate pressure, and checking for sensitivity, which may indicate an issue in the associated body part. Consistency in recognizing and understanding these zones will significantly enhance your ability to target reflex points accurately and promote healing.

Foot, Hand, And Ear Reflex Maps

Foot reflex maps are foundational in reflexology, showing which areas of the feet correspond to organs and systems in the body.

For example, the toes are connected to the head, and the arch of the foot correlates with digestive organs like the stomach and intestines.

Practicing on the feet provides a broad approach, addressing numerous body parts through carefully mapped zones.

Hand reflex maps serve as an accessible alternative to foot reflexology, especially in settings where removing shoes is impractical.

Each finger corresponds to parts of the head, while the palms reflect the body's central organs. Using a hand map, you can easily stimulate the stomach, heart, and spine reflex points simply by applying gentle pressure to the center of the palm and moving outward.

Ear reflex maps are also effective, often used to stimulate immediate relaxation. The ear's structure has zones that mirror the entire body in a curled, fetal-like position, meaning the earlobe corresponds to the head, while the upper ear connects to the lower body.

Gentle circular motions along the ear can activate these zones, especially beneficial when quick stress relief is needed.

Key Reflex Points For Common Ailments
For headaches, you can focus on the reflex points at the tips of the toes (for feet) or fingertips (for hands), as these areas correlate with the head and brain.

Press and release gently, massaging each point for a few seconds. Repeating this action for two to three minutes can often relieve tension, making it a helpful remedy for mild headaches.

Digestive issues can be targeted through the arch of the foot, which corresponds to the stomach, intestines, and other digestive organs.

Use your thumbs to apply rolling pressure along the inner arch, starting from the heel to the ball of the foot. This can help stimulate digestion and alleviate issues like bloating or indigestion.

For fatigue or low energy, the reflex point for the adrenal glands, located on the center of the balls of the feet or the fleshy part below the thumb on the hands, is ideal. Firmly press and massage this point for a few seconds at a time to boost vitality. Practicing this daily can be particularly effective for reducing stress and rejuvenating energy levels.

The Concept Of Energy Zones

Energy zones are imaginary lines that run vertically from head to toe, dividing the body into five zones on each side, creating mirrored zones on the left and right. Each zone has reflex points on the corresponding foot, hand, and ear.

Understanding these zones can help you target reflex points with accuracy, enhancing the effectiveness of your practice.

The zones influence the body's flow of energy, so if there's discomfort or imbalance in one zone, it may signal an issue with the organ or body part within that area. For instance, if there's pain in Zone 1, the area from your head to your big toe, it might point to issues along the spine or digestive tract, both of which align with Zone 1.

To apply energy zone concepts in reflexology, locate the problem area on the foot, hand, or ear, and begin by stimulating reflex points within the same zone. This approach ensures that all interconnected parts receive equal attention, promoting balance and optimal health throughout the body.

Tips For Locating Reflex Points Accurately

Accurately locating reflex points is essential for effective reflexology practice. Start by familiarizing yourself with reflex maps and studying where specific points correspond to organs. Use your fingers or thumbs to lightly press each area, feeling for tenderness, as this often signals an active reflex point in need of attention.

Keep a steady, gentle pressure on the targeted point, applying circular or rolling motions for best results. Avoid pressing too hard; sensitivity varies between individuals, so adjusting pressure to comfort levels ensures a better experience. Start with the main zones and work gradually in other areas to build your skills.

To make locating reflex points easier, use a small tool like a rounded stick or reflexology wand, which allows more precision. Practicing consistently will not only improve your reflex location skills but also build your intuition on which areas need focus. Eventually, with patience and practice, you'll recognize reflex points naturally.

Importance Of Consistency In Practice
Consistency is key in reflexology, as a regular practice helps reinforce the connection

between reflex points and their corresponding body parts. By stimulating these points daily or weekly, you promote blood circulation, reduce stress, and support overall balance. Regular sessions also make you more attuned to your body, allowing you to detect potential health issues early.

Maintaining a consistent schedule allows your body to reap the cumulative benefits of reflexology. It's ideal to start with short, frequent sessions and gradually extend the time as you become more comfortable. Aim for at least 15 minutes per session, focusing on specific areas that may need extra attention.

Consistency also builds confidence and intuition, helping you understands which areas respond best to pressure. Over time, you'll learn to adapt your technique based on your body's feedback, making each session more effective.

This long-term commitment can foster a sense of control over your wellness, reinforcing reflexology as a self-care tool.

CHAPTER THREE

Essential Techniques For Beginners

In reflexology, understanding the core techniques is key to effectively stimulating various points on the feet and hands that correspond to different areas of the body. For beginners, it's helpful to start by learning how to identify reflex zones. These are specific areas of the feet and hands that, when massaged, influence related organs and systems. A simple way to begin is by gently pressing each area, noting any areas that feel particularly tense or tender.

Next, practice "walking" with your thumb or fingers over these reflex zones. To do this, hold the foot or hand with one hand while the other hand moves in small steps with the thumb or fingers. This motion helps beginners get comfortable with navigating the different reflex areas without overstimulating any one point. Try covering the entire foot or hand in this way to become familiar with each zone.

Another essential technique for beginners is learning to sense and respond to the body's feedback. Reflexology isn't about applying heavy pressure but rather about finding balance. If a person feels pain or discomfort, ease the pressure slightly and continue with gentle movements. This technique helps you gauge how much pressure each area can handle and provides a more comfortable experience for the person receiving the reflexology session.

Basic Thumb And Finger Techniques

Thumb and finger techniques are fundamental to reflexology. The "thumb walking" technique involves bending the thumb at each joint as you move it across the foot or hand, creating a motion that allows for consistent pressure. To try it, hold the foot or hand steady and press with the thumb, lifting and lowering it as you "walk" along each area. This technique can be repeated over the same spot a few times to address tension points.

Another effective method is the "finger walking" technique, which is especially useful for smaller or more sensitive areas like the toes and fingers. Use the pads of your fingers to create a similar walking motion, pressing down with each finger and releasing rhythmically. This technique can provide a more nuanced approach for areas that may require lighter pressure.

The "hook and back-up" technique is another useful method where the thumb or finger applies pressure in a hooking motion, slightly pulling back after each press. This is beneficial for areas that feel particularly tight or need deeper stimulation. Beginners should practice each of these techniques to get a feel for how each affects different parts of the feet and hands and to build comfort and skill.

Applying Appropriate Pressure

Knowing how much pressure to apply is essential in reflexology, as the wrong amount can cause discomfort or reduce the technique's effectiveness.

Start with light to medium pressure when working with reflex zones, adjusting as needed based on the person's comfort level. A good rule is to observe their responses; if they wince or tense up, it's a signal to reduce the pressure.

For sensitive areas, such as near the toes or around the inner foot, use your thumb or fingers with minimal pressure, focusing on a gentle, controlled motion. Heavier pressure can be used on tougher areas like the heels or arches, but only if the person finds it comfortable.

Practice maintaining a balance between firmness and gentleness to avoid overworking any single area.

Finally, applying appropriate pressure involves paying attention to the rhythm of your movements. Steady, moderate pressure with rhythmic motions helps create a relaxing experience and enhances the effectiveness of each reflexology session. This rhythm allows the person's muscles and nerves to adapt to the pressure, promoting a deeper sense of relaxation without overstimulation.

Common Mistakes And How To Avoid Them

A common mistake for beginners is applying too much pressure, which can lead to discomfort or even minor injuries. Always start with light pressure and adjust gradually. Reflexology should feel soothing, not painful; discomfort is a signal that the pressure is too strong.

Avoiding heavy pressure also ensures that sensitive areas are treated with care, making for a more enjoyable session.

Another mistake is neglecting to warm up the hands or feet before beginning the session. Cold muscles are more likely to feel sore or tight, so it's important to warm up the area first by gently massaging each section. A basic warm-up can make the entire experience smoother and more comfortable, as it relaxes the muscles and prepares them for deeper pressure.

Failing to cover all reflex zones evenly is also a common oversight. Beginners may spend too much time on one area and miss others, leading to an imbalanced session.

Make it a habit to work through the whole foot or hand methodically, using thumb or finger techniques. This ensures comprehensive coverage and maximizes the health benefits associated with reflexology.

Techniques For Relaxing And Warming Up

Starting a reflexology session with relaxing and warming-up techniques helps ease the person into a calm state. Begin by gently holding the foot or hand, allowing them to relax as you apply light pressure with both hands.

Use a few moments here to create a peaceful atmosphere, letting them adjust to the touch and preparing the muscles for deeper work.

Once comfortable, use gentle circular motions around the ankles or wrists to increase blood flow. This loosens up the entire area and helps ease any stiffness in the joints. Follow this by "kneading" the larger areas of the foot or hand, pressing down with your thumb and palm in gentle, sweeping motions. This technique further warms the muscles, making them more receptive to the reflexology session.

Incorporating breathing techniques with the person receiving reflexology can enhance relaxation. Encourage slow, deep breathing to help them relax while you begin applying gentle, rhythmic pressure. This helps create a calming environment, where they feel at ease, leading to a more successful and enjoyable reflexology session.

Safety Tips For Effective Sessions

Safety is a priority in reflexology, as the goal is to promote health and relaxation without causing strain. Always check for any existing injuries or conditions that could make reflexology painful or risky. For example, if someone has plantar fasciitis or any foot condition, apply extra care and avoid heavy pressure on those areas.

Hygiene is equally important to ensure a safe and comfortable experience. Wash and dry your hands thoroughly before and after each session, and if needed, use a light, non-greasy lotion to keep the skin from becoming irritated during the session.

Clean, warm hands also help create a more relaxing experience for the person receiving reflexology.

In addition, ensure that your posture is comfortable to avoid straining your own body. Sitting in a stable position allows you to apply controlled pressure without straining your back or wrists. Safety in reflexology is about creating a balanced, mindful approach, where both the practitioner and recipient feel comfortable and supported throughout the session.

CHAPTER FOUR

Step-By-Step Foot Reflexology

To start foot reflexology, have the recipient seated or lying down with feet comfortably exposed. Start with a gentle warm-up by lightly pressing and rubbing both feet, focusing on the arch, heel, and toes. This helps increase circulation and relaxes the muscles, preparing them for deeper work. Use your thumbs to apply firm yet gentle pressure, moving from the heel up to the toes in a slow, rolling motion.

After warming up, move to specific zones on each foot, each corresponding to different body systems. For example, press on the big toe to stimulate the brain and sinuses. Next, apply pressure to the ball of the foot, linked to the lungs and chest. Move to the arch to target digestive organs like the stomach and intestines. Gently press on each point for about 3-5 seconds, using a thumb-walking motion to go deeper without causing discomfort.

End the session by massaging the entire foot, making gentle circles on the top and bottom to release any lingering tension. Gently squeeze each toe and pull lightly to stretch the tendons.

Finish with a light, soothing rub across the foot to leave the recipient feeling calm and rejuvenated. Repeat on the other foot to ensure balanced relaxation throughout the body.

Preparing The Feet For Reflexology

Start by washing and drying the feet thoroughly to ensure they're clean and free of any oils or lotions that may cause slipping during the session. Next, sit in a comfortable position with your foot elevated on a soft surface or pillow, which helps relieve any strain. A quick soak in warm water with a few drops of essential oils, like lavender or eucalyptus, can also help relax the muscles and soothe the skin.

Once the feet are dry, massage a small amount of unscented lotion or oil onto each foot to keep the skin hydrated and enhance the flow of reflexology movements. Use light strokes to spread the lotion evenly, covering areas from the heel to the toes. This preparatory massage helps release tension and boosts circulation, making it easier to feel specific reflex points during the session.

To check for sensitive spots, gently press different areas on the foot using your thumb. If any area feels tender, spend a bit more time massaging it to release any knots or tension. This step prepares the foot for more targeted reflexology work and ensures a smooth, effective session for both the giver and receiver.

Key Reflex Points On The Feet And Their Benefits

The big toe represents the head and brain, and pressing on this area helps clear the mind and alleviate headaches. The inner edge of the big toe relates to the spine, so gently pressing along this area can relieve back tension. Massaging the top half of the big toe can stimulate the pituitary gland, promoting hormonal balance.

The ball of the foot is connected to the chest and lung region. Firmly pressing this area can help improve breathing and relieve chest tightness. Moving to the arch, which is linked to the digestive system, gentle pressure here can support stomach health, alleviate bloating, and relieve digestive discomfort. Pressing on this area may also aid in stress reduction due to its close connection with the adrenal glands.

Finally, the heel and ankle are linked to the lower body, especially reproductive organs and the sciatic nerve.

Gently pressing and massaging the heel can relieve hip and lower back pain. Exploring these key reflex points with consistent, gentle pressure can promote a sense of balance and relaxation throughout the body, enhancing overall well-being.

Foot Reflexology Techniques For Beginners

Beginner reflexologists should start with the "thumb-walking" technique, where you walk your thumb in small steps along the foot. Hold the foot with one hand, using your thumb to apply light pressure in a straight line, moving gradually across the foot.

This technique allows you to explore reflex points while applying controlled pressure that's comfortable for the recipient.

Next, try the "finger rotation" technique. Gently press down on a point, then rotate your thumb or finger in small circles while maintaining consistent pressure.

This method is great for working on specific areas that may feel tight, as the circular motion helps release tension effectively. Use this on the arch or heel for better results with digestive and reproductive organ reflex points.

For relaxation, use the "caterpillar" technique by curling and uncurling your fingers in a wave-like motion along the sides of the foot. This provides a soothing touch that helps release stress and eases into more intense reflexology points.

Practicing these techniques can help beginners gain confidence in identifying key points and applying effective reflexology methods.

How To Sequence Foot Reflexology Steps

Start by warming up the foot, which prepares the muscles and reflex points. Use soft, stroking motions from the heel to the toes to stimulate blood flow and gently loosen tight muscles. Then move on to the toes, beginning with the big toe and working down to the smaller ones, pressing gently to stimulate the brain and sinus reflex points.

Continue to the ball of the foot to address reflexes related to the lungs and chest. Apply steady pressure here before moving to the arch, which corresponds to the digestive organs. Spend extra time on any areas that feel tense, using a thumb-walking motion. After this, move to the heel to stimulate lower body reflexes, including those for the sciatic nerve and reproductive organs.

Finish by giving the entire foot a soothing massage, using gentle circular motions to wrap up the session. Make sure to work both feet in the same sequence for balance. This organized sequence promotes a full-body relaxation effect and allows each reflex area to be thoroughly stimulated, enhancing the benefits of foot reflexology.

Tips For Self-Reflexology On The Feet
For a self-reflexology session, start by sitting in a comfortable chair and lifting one foot

onto your opposite thigh. This position lets you easily reach all areas of the foot.

Use your thumb to apply gentle pressure, starting with the toes and working down to the heel. Breathe deeply, as this promotes relaxation and focus on the process.

Focus on key areas like the arch, where the digestive system reflexes are located, by pressing gently and moving your thumb in circular motions. For added relaxation, massage the ball of your foot, which connects to the lungs, to deepen your breathing. The heel is also a key point; pressing here helps with lower back tension and releases stress from the hips and legs.

You can even use small tools like a reflexology stick or rubber ball for deeper pressure on specific areas. Roll the ball under your foot for 2-3 minutes, focusing on tense areas.

Self-reflexology can be a powerful relaxation tool that's easy to integrate into your routine. Just 10–15 minutes a few times a week can leave you feeling rejuvenated.

CHAPTER FIVE

Hand Reflexology Basics

Hand reflexology is a therapeutic technique that involves applying pressure to specific points on the hands that correspond to different organs and systems in the body. By stimulating these points, practitioners believe it can help alleviate pain, reduce stress, and promote overall well-being. The hands contain a map of the body, with each part of the hand linking to specific areas, organs, or functions. This non-invasive technique is easy to perform, making it suitable for self-care or as a part of holistic health practices.

To get started with hand reflexology, all you need is a quiet place and a few minutes to focus on each hand. Sit comfortably, use your thumb or fingers to apply pressure to various areas, and take deep breaths to enhance relaxation. Practitioners recommend starting with light to moderate pressure and observing how your body responds. As you gain confidence, you can increase the pressure to better stimulate each reflex point.

Hand reflexology can be practiced anytime, whether you're at home, at work, or on a break. Since it's highly adaptable, it doesn't require specialized equipment.

Beginners can easily learn to locate reflex points with simple charts or illustrations, helping them understand which points to press for specific benefits like headache relief, digestion support, or sleep improvement.

Advantages Of Hand Reflexology

Hand reflexology offers various physical, emotional, and mental health benefits, making it a valuable addition to any wellness routine.

It's often used to relieve tension and promote relaxation by reducing cortisol levels and soothing nervous tension. By targeting reflex points associated with stress relief, individuals can help alleviate everyday anxiety, improve mood, and enhance resilience to stress over time.

Aside from emotional benefits, hand reflexology can support pain management, especially for issues like headaches, neck tension, or arthritis-related discomfort. Reflex points connected to the spine, head, and joints, when gently stimulated, can help alleviate aches and improve circulation. For those with digestive issues, stimulating reflexes related to the stomach and intestines can encourage better digestion and reduce bloating.

Hand reflexology is also practical because of its accessibility. Unlike full-body reflexology, it can be done quickly and discreetly, allowing people to address health issues on the go. This flexibility makes it easy to integrate into daily life, even during busy schedules, helping individuals feel balanced, focused, and energized throughout the day.

Key Reflex Points On The Hands

The hands contain several reflex points linked to major organs and body functions, making it easy to target specific issues.

The thumb is a primary reflex point for the brain and head, making it a good place to start if you're experiencing headaches or mental fatigue. The base of the thumb and the inner area of the wrist correspond to the lungs and chest, which can help stimulate during respiratory discomfort or stress.

Another key point is the center of the palm, which is associated with the stomach and digestive system. Gently pressing this area may help alleviate digestive discomfort, bloating, and stomach cramps. For those with back pain, the area along the outer edge of the hand (from the pinky to the wrist) represents the spine. Applying light pressure here can help soothe spinal tension and improve posture-related discomfort.

The fingers are connected to sinus and eye health, which can be helpful during allergy season or when experiencing eye strain. By understanding these points, you can effectively address specific health concerns. Using a reflexology chart as a guide is beneficial for beginners to locate points accurately and maximize the benefits of this practice.

Basic Hand Reflexology Techniques

Starting with a warm-up technique, rub your hands together for a few seconds to activate energy and improve circulation. Next, use your thumb to apply steady, circular pressure to each reflex point, holding for 5-10 seconds before moving on. For beginners, it's best to apply gentle pressure and gradually increase intensity based on comfort.

Another effective technique is the thumb-walking method, where you move your thumb in a 'walking' motion along specific points on the hands. This allows you to target reflex zones with controlled pressure, moving from one area to another seamlessly. Thumb-walking is particularly effective along the spine reflex area on the outer edge of the hand and helps alleviate back and neck tension.

Finally, try using finger-pinching on the tips of each finger, which can help with sinus relief and stimulate the nervous system. This technique is simple but impactful, especially for relieving sinus headaches or eye strain.

Practice each technique on both hands and remember to breathe deeply to enhance relaxation and improve energy flow.

Best Practices For Self-Hand Reflexology
For effective self-hand reflexology, start by finding a comfortable and quiet place where you can focus. Use a reflexology chart to familiarize yourself with the key points before beginning.

To maximize the benefits, begin with gentle warm-up exercises, like rotating your wrists or rubbing your hands together to relax the muscles and increase circulation.

During the session, try to be mindful of how much pressure you apply. Always start with light pressure and gradually increase as needed to avoid any discomfort or soreness.

Ensure that you're not pressing too hard, especially on sensitive areas, and take breaks between reflex points if needed. Practicing mindfulness during the process will help you notice the positive effects more clearly.

Incorporate breathing exercises to enhance relaxation while pressing each point. Breathing deeply and evenly helps activate the body's relaxation response, amplifying the therapeutic effects of reflexology.

Additionally, staying consistent with your practice will make it more effective over time, helping you recognize which techniques and pressure points work best for your body.

Integrating Hand Reflexology Into Daily Routines

To integrate hand reflexology into daily life, set aside a few minutes each day for a mini-session, whether in the morning, midday, or before bed. For example, pressing the brain reflex point on the thumb each morning can improve focus and mental clarity for the day ahead. Use reflexology as a quick break at work to relieve stress by pressing points linked to relaxation and emotional well-being.

You can also use hand reflexology as part of your evening routine by focusing on reflex points that help promote sleep, like the stomach and head reflexes. A short session before bed can help relieve digestive issues and calm your mind, preparing you for a restful sleep.

Practicing reflexology in the evening can be especially beneficial if you experience stress-related insomnia.

Incorporating hand reflexology into daily life doesn't require large time commitments; even short sessions can make a difference. Practicing reflexology while watching TV, commuting, or on a break makes it easy to adopt without disrupting your schedule. This regularity will help reinforce the benefits, making hand reflexology a natural part of your wellness routine.

CHAPTER SIX

Ear Reflexology For Quick Relief

Introduction To Auricular (Ear) Reflexology

Ear reflexology is a therapeutic technique based on the principle that specific points on the ear correspond to different parts of the body. Applying pressure to these areas stimulates nerves and promotes natural healing by balancing the nervous system. It is a holistic approach to health, often used to relieve stress, headaches, anxiety, and chronic pain.

Unlike traditional foot or hand reflexology, ear reflexology can be performed discreetly, offering quick relief anywhere, anytime.

This practice stems from both ancient Chinese medicine and modern discoveries. French neurologist Dr. Paul Nogier popularized auricular therapy by mapping out reflex points on the ear that connect with the nervous system. Practitioners view the ear as a microcosm of the body, similar to how reflex zones on the feet or hands reflect internal systems. It's particularly effective for addressing immediate concerns like nausea or pain without requiring elaborate tools.

The beauty of ear reflexology lies in its simplicity: all you need is knowledge of the key points and your fingers, or occasionally a blunt tool like an eraser end. Whether done by a professional or self-administered, it's a flexible and powerful method for promoting wellness.

Key Reflex Points On The Ears

Several critical reflex points are found in the ear. The Shen Men (or "Heavenly Gate") is one of the most powerful points, located at the upper-central part of the ear. It helps reduce stress, alleviate pain, and boost relaxation. The ear lobe contains reflex points that correspond to the head and face, which makes it effective for headache relief or sinus issues.

The Anti-Helix curve reflects the spine and joints, making it a useful target for relieving back or neck tension. Additionally, the Triangular Fossa, a small indentation near the upper-middle ear, corresponds to the pelvic organs and is frequently used to ease menstrual pain or urinary issues. Knowing these key areas makes ear reflexology precise and impactful.

Mapping out the ear may seem complex at first, but most practitioners recommend starting with basic, accessible points. You can even experiment by gently massaging the ear lobe or Shen Men area for a few minutes to notice how your body responds. With time and practice, recognizing these reflex points becomes second nature.

Simple Techniques For Ear Reflexology

Start by sitting comfortably in a quiet environment. Begin by warming up the ear by rubbing it gently between your fingers. This increases blood flow and prepares the ear for deeper work.

Then, locate your desired reflex point—say, the Shen Men—using your thumb and index finger to apply firm but comfortable pressure. Hold for 30-60 seconds, or until you feel slight warmth or tingling.

You can also use circular motions to massage the point, which further stimulates nerve endings. Some people find that applying light pressure in rhythm with their breathing enhances relaxation. If using tools, ensure they are rounded and smooth to avoid discomfort or injury.

Try to perform ear reflexology regularly—either as a daily routine or as needed for quick relief. It's especially useful to practice during moments of stress or discomfort. The portability of this method means you can do it discreetly at work, on public transport, or before bed for a relaxing wind-down.

Common Issues Treated With Ear Reflexology

Ear reflexology is known for alleviating a wide range of conditions. For stress and anxiety, massaging the Shen Men or the Sympathetic Autonomic Point can provide almost immediate relief. Headaches and migraines can be addressed by applying pressure to the ear lobe or the Temple point.

It is also beneficial for managing digestive issues such as nausea and bloating. By stimulating the Digestive Reflex point located on the ear's outer ridge, symptoms can often be eased. Additionally, reflex points linked to the spine and joints can help alleviate muscle tension, stiffness, and chronic pain in the back or neck.

Some practitioners use ear reflexology as part of a holistic treatment plan for insomnia, menstrual pain, and even addiction management. By stimulating the right reflex points, many individuals experience long-term improvements in their overall well-being.

Cautions And Limitations With Ear Reflexology

Although ear reflexology is generally safe, certain precautions should be taken. Pregnant individuals should consult a healthcare professional before starting reflexology, as some points may induce contractions. Similarly, those with existing ear infections or injuries should avoid manipulating the ear until fully healed.

If you experience discomfort or dizziness while performing reflexology, stop immediately and rest. Avoid using sharp objects or excessive force to prevent injury. Ear reflexology is meant to be gentle and soothing—pressing too hard can cause unnecessary pain.

While ear reflexology offers effective relief for many ailments, it is not a substitute for professional medical care. It works best as a complementary therapy alongside conventional treatments, particularly for chronic conditions. Always consult with your doctor for serious medical concerns.

CHAPTER SEVEN

Reflexology For Stress Relief And Relaxation

Reflexology offers a natural method to alleviate stress, using targeted pressure points on the feet, hands, and sometimes ears to promote relaxation. Stress relief through reflexology often begins with gentle circular motions applied to the soles of the feet or palms of the hands, helping to ease muscle tension and create a sense of calm. Practitioners typically start by warming up the hands and feet, allowing for a smooth transition into the session and creating a calm atmosphere that promotes relaxation.

Key reflex points for stress relief include the solar plexus reflex, found in the center of the foot's arch, and points on the toes that correlate with the head and mind. To activate these, apply gentle pressure with your thumb or fingers, moving in small circles or by pressing and releasing. These techniques help reduce tension and encourage deep relaxation, making it easier for the body to enter a state of rest and repair.

To maintain effectiveness, consistent reflexology sessions—either weekly or biweekly—are recommended. Self-practice can also be beneficial, focusing on pressing areas like the tops of the toes and soles of the feet whenever you feel stressed. This practice helps release pent-up stress and improve blood circulation, aiding in an overall calmer state.

Understanding How Reflexology Reduces Stress

Reflexology targets specific nerve endings that correspond to various organs and body parts, helping to manage stress by balancing these systems. Stress disrupts natural body rhythms, but reflexology aims to restore these rhythms by improving circulation and promoting relaxation through gentle, targeted pressure. By working on reflex points connected to the central nervous system, reflexology facilitates the release of endorphins, reducing stress hormones and fostering a feeling of well-being.

The practice encourages the parasympathetic nervous system to engage, helping the body naturally calm down and recover from stress.

For example, applying pressure to the area of the foot associated with the brain and neck can ease headaches and reduce muscle tension. Reflexologists often use techniques like thumb-walking to cover all areas systematically, ensuring that every reflex point connected to stress relief is stimulated.

Reflexology is not just about immediate stress reduction; it's also preventative. Regular sessions help lower baseline stress levels, improving mental resilience over time. Many people incorporate reflexology into their wellness routine because of its cumulative benefits, as it helps balance the body's natural energy pathways, reduces stress, and creates lasting mental clarity and calm.

Calming Reflex Points For Anxiety

Certain reflex points are particularly effective for relieving anxiety, often located on the feet, hands, and ears. The solar plexus reflex, located in the center of each foot's arch, is one of the most effective points for immediate anxiety relief. Gently pressing this area with the thumb while breathing slowly can help reduce anxiety symptoms quickly. Practitioners often start a session by applying pressure to this point, as it has a grounding effect.

Another important point is the adrenal reflex, found below the ball of each foot. By pressing here, you can help regulate stress hormones, especially adrenaline, which is often elevated in anxious individuals.

To activate this, apply firm yet comfortable pressure with your thumb in a circular motion, pausing to breathe deeply as you work through each foot.

For additional anxiety relief, try massaging the points on the tips of your fingers or toes, which connect to the head and mind. This can help alleviate racing thoughts and mental tension. Taking time each day to focus on these areas in a quiet setting allows for both immediate and long-term anxiety reduction, making it a powerful tool for anyone managing anxiety.

Creating A Relaxing Environment For Sessions

Setting up a calming environment is essential for a successful reflexology session, as it helps both the practitioner and recipient feel at ease. Begin by choosing a quiet, clutter-free area, and add soft lighting to enhance relaxation. Incorporate elements like candles, essential oils, or incense to create a soothing atmosphere that helps you fully relax into the experience.

Use comfortable seating or a recliner where you can easily access your feet or hands. For added comfort, lay down a soft towel and place a warm compress on the feet before beginning the session. Background music, like calming instrumentals or nature sounds, can also be beneficial. These sensory additions can enhance the experience, creating a sanctuary-like atmosphere that promotes relaxation.

Practitioners can also incorporate grounding techniques, like taking a few deep breaths together at the start of the session. This not only sets the tone but helps you connect to the present moment, reducing distractions and creating a positive mental space. Having a dedicated, calming environment greatly enhances reflexology's relaxation benefits, making each session more effective.

Using Reflexology For Better Sleep

Reflexology is an excellent tool for improving sleep, as it can help relieve both physical and mental tension that often disrupts sleep. By focusing on reflex points connected to the nervous system and brain, reflexology encourages the body to enter a deeper state of relaxation, which is essential for restful sleep. The best time to use reflexology for sleep is in the evening, as it helps release any built-up stress from the day.

Key areas for sleep improvement include the big toe, which is associated with the brain and pineal gland, responsible for regulating sleep cycles. Gently massaging the big toe with small, circular motions or holding pressure can help stimulate melatonin production, aiding in the onset of sleep. Another effective point is the area between the arches, which can relieve tension and encourage relaxation of the entire body.

Incorporating reflexology into a nightly routine can make a noticeable difference in sleep quality over time. Consistent practice helps align the body's internal clock, reducing insomnia and other sleep disturbances. Self-massage techniques before bed can become a comforting ritual that signals to your body that it's time to wind down and prepare for deep, restful sleep.

Tips For Maximizing Relaxation Benefits
To get the most from reflexology, consider incorporating relaxation techniques like deep breathing and mindfulness during your session. Start each reflexology session by taking a few deep breaths to clear your mind and bring attention to your body. This primes your nervous system to relax and helps each reflex point you work on to respond more effectively.

In addition to proper technique, focus on regularity. Practicing reflexology consistently, even for a few minutes each day, can accumulate significant relaxation benefits. Aim for at least 10 to 15 minutes per session, targeting specific points that correspond with relaxation or stress relief. Adding gentle stretching afterward can also aid in relaxing the muscles and prolonging the feeling of calm.

Lastly, drink water after each session to help flush out toxins and improve the body's recovery. Staying hydrated is essential for the relaxation benefits to take full effect. Over time, these small practices contribute to greater mental clarity, improved relaxation, and a healthier stress response system, making reflexology a key part of a holistic wellness routine.

CHAPTER EIGHT

Reflexology For Pain Management And Healing

Reflexology for pain management involves stimulating specific points on the feet, hands, or ears that correspond to different parts of the body. By applying gentle, targeted pressure, reflexology helps release tension, promote relaxation, and improve blood flow, which can lead to reduced pain levels.

Reflexologists often use thumb-walking techniques, gentle tapping, or circular motions to stimulate these reflex points. To alleviate general pain, try pressing on the tops and sides of the toes and fingers, which are linked to the head and upper body.

To enhance the healing process, reflexology encourages the body's natural energy flow, believed to activate its self-healing abilities. During a session, you may start by warming up the entire foot or hand with light strokes. Reflex points on the arch of the foot, in particular, connect to the spine and can be pressed to relieve stress along the back, helping with overall body alignment. Practitioners may also focus on areas connected to the immune system, such as points on the big toes, to promote recovery from injuries or illness.

For those with chronic pain, regular reflexology sessions can provide long-term relief by reducing inflammation and relaxing tense muscles.

Establishing a routine of gentle, targeted foot massages once or twice a week can make a significant difference. If doing this at home, remember to maintain a firm but comfortable pressure and take breaks to allow the body to adjust. Reflexology's non-invasive approach makes it accessible to most people and adaptable to individual pain thresholds and sensitivity.

Identifying Reflex Points For Pain Relief
Identifying reflex points is key to effective reflexology, as each point on the hands, feet, and ears correlates with specific organs, muscles, and bodily systems. To locate the reflex points for pain relief, start by dividing the feet or hands into sections, typically the toes/fingers for the head and neck, the middle

for the torso and organs, and the heels for the lower body and pelvic areas. Using a reflexology chart can help you pinpoint the exact areas associated with your discomfort.

For example, if you have headaches, focus on the reflex points on the big toe, which correspond to the head. For stomach or digestive issues, the inner arch area of the foot may offer relief. To ease back pain, work along the length of the inner foot arch, which mirrors the spine. Apply gentle pressure to these points with your thumb or fingers, using a rolling motion, and spend a few seconds on each area to identify spots that feel tender, as this often indicates an area needing attention.

Once you identify these reflex points, create a routine to address specific types of pain consistently. You may find some areas to be more sensitive; these could be signs that they need extra care. Use a gradual increase in pressure as you get used to the sensation, and ensure you practice on both feet or hands to maintain balance in your body's energy and response.

Techniques For Headache And Migraine Relief

To relieve headaches and migraines using reflexology, focus on stimulating reflex points on the feet and hands connected to the head and neck. Begin by applying gentle pressure to the big toes and fingertips, specifically the tips and outer edges. A circular motion in these areas can reduce tension around the temples and forehead, which often contributes to headache pain.

Next, target the area between the toes on both feet, which relates to the lymphatic system and can help relieve sinus pressure, a common migraine trigger. Reflexologists often recommend the "pinch and release" technique for headache relief, where you gently pinch the outer edge of the big toe and then let go. This action helps to release energy blockages that may be causing discomfort. You can also press firmly on the middle of the thumb pad for a minute or so, as this area corresponds to the head and sinuses.

For maximum effect, combine reflexology with deep breathing exercises to encourage full-body relaxation. Practicing a few deep, slow breaths while stimulating these points can enhance the release of tension and stress.

This technique can be especially beneficial for migraines, as it addresses both the physical and emotional triggers of pain, encouraging a calm, focused mind.

Reflexology For Back And Joint Pain

Reflexology can help relieve back and joint pain by targeting the inner edge of the feet and hands, which corresponds to the spine and surrounding muscle groups. Begin by applying light to moderate pressure along the inner arch of the foot, using your thumb to make small, circular motions from the heel to the base of the toes. This area reflects the entire spinal column, and working here can help ease tension in the back.

For joint pain, reflexologists often focus on the toes and fingers, which are connected to the body's main joints. Pressing on the toe joints and knuckles can help relieve discomfort in the knees, hips, shoulders, and other areas. Use a combination of steady pressure and gentle stroking on these points, adjusting the intensity as needed. Regular practice on these reflex points can reduce joint stiffness and improve flexibility over time.

For targeted relief, repeat the process on both feet or hands several times, focusing on particularly sensitive areas. Practicing reflexology in warm water or after a warm foot bath can be especially effective, as heat helps relax muscles and increases blood flow, making the process more soothing and beneficial for back and joint pain.

Managing Digestive Discomfort With Reflexology

Reflexology is useful for managing digestive issues by focusing on points linked to the stomach, intestines, and other digestive organs, which are located mainly on the inner arches of the feet and palms. To begin, start with gentle stroking on the middle area of the foot's inner arch, which corresponds to the stomach, spleen, and intestines. This area can relieve symptoms of indigestion and bloating when stimulated gently.

To alleviate nausea or stomach cramps, use circular motions on the upper middle section of the foot, as this area connects to the stomach. The lower arch, closer to the heel, is linked to the lower digestive tract, and pressing here can help with bowel regularity.

Reflexologists may suggest rotating your thumb in this area for a few seconds before moving to the other foot to stimulate a balanced effect across both sides.

To complete the digestive routine, press on the center of the sole, just below the ball of the foot, which corresponds to the solar plexus and can help relieve stress that often impacts digestion? Practicing these techniques consistently can improve digestive comfort, particularly when used alongside a healthy diet and hydration practices.

Using Reflexology For Improved Circulation

Reflexology improves circulation by stimulating points on the feet and hands that promote blood flow, helping oxygen and nutrients reach vital organs more efficiently. To enhance circulation, focus on the balls of the feet, pressing gently in an upward and outward motion. This area relates to the heart and lungs, and stimulating it encourages better blood and oxygen flow.

The toes are another key area to target, as each corresponds to the body's upper circulation points. Begin by lightly pinching and massaging each toe, starting from the big toe and moving outward, which can help relieve cold extremities. Use your thumbs to press down on the base of each toe to further encourage blood flow to the hands, feet, and other extremities, helping with both circulation and relaxation.

For a complete circulation routine, finish with gentle stroking from the heel to the toes, as this activates the whole foot and energizes the circulatory system. Regular practice, combined with deep breathing exercises, can make a noticeable difference for anyone with circulation issues, as reflexology supports overall cardiovascular health naturally and gently.

CHAPTER NINE

Common Concerns And Questions In Reflexology

Many people new to reflexology wonder about its purpose and benefits. Reflexology is a therapy focusing on applying pressure to specific points on the feet, hands, or ears, which are believed to correspond to various body organs and systems. The technique is meant to relieve stress, enhance relaxation, and improve overall wellness. Reflexology can aid in reducing headaches, improving digestion, and helping with insomnia, among other potential benefits.

A common question is whether reflexology is painful. Reflexology is generally a gentle technique, but some areas may feel tender, especially if there's tension in the corresponding body part. Practitioners often adjust their pressure to match individual comfort levels, and any discomfort typically lessens with regular sessions. Reflexology should feel relaxing and restorative, leaving clients with a sense of calm and well-being.

Another frequent concern is how long it takes to notice benefits. Some people experience immediate relaxation or reduced stress, while others may require several sessions to see improvement in specific areas. Responses to reflexology vary widely, and while it's not a guaranteed solution for medical issues, many find it a beneficial complementary therapy. Practicing patience and consistency can maximize the benefits over time.

Is Reflexology Safe For Everyone?

Reflexology is generally considered safe for most people, as it's non-invasive and doesn't involve medication or manipulations. For the majority, reflexology promotes relaxation and can be a great tool for managing stress. However, certain groups may need to take precautions, including pregnant women, individuals with circulatory issues, and people with severe foot injuries or infections.

Pregnant women should consult their healthcare provider before trying reflexology, as some reflex points are believed to influence reproductive organs. Reflexology can be beneficial during pregnancy for relieving stress and minor discomforts, but it's best to work with a therapist experienced in prenatal reflexology to avoid any potential risks. Similarly, people with recent surgeries, blood clotting disorders, or severe circulatory issues should consult a healthcare professional before beginning reflexology.

If you have health concerns, discuss them openly with your reflexologist before starting. A professional reflexologist will adjust pressure and avoid sensitive areas as needed. Ultimately, reflexology's safety largely depends on the practitioner's skill, so finding a trained and certified reflexologist can ensure a comfortable, safe experience.

Reflexology Vs. Massage: Key Differences

While both reflexology and massage promote relaxation and wellness, they are distinct therapies with different techniques and goals. Reflexology focuses on applying pressure to specific reflex points on the feet, hands, and ears to stimulate body functions and promote energy flow. Each point is believed to correspond to an organ or system, making reflexology a more targeted therapy.

Massage, on the other hand, involves manipulating larger muscle groups throughout the body to relieve tension, improve circulation, and release physical stress.

Massage therapists use kneading, pressing, and rubbing techniques on muscles and soft tissues, while reflexology focuses on smaller, precise pressure points. Massage is more about physical muscle relaxation, whereas reflexology aims to support holistic wellness through energy channels.

Another key difference lies in the treatment experience. Reflexology sessions often take place fully clothed (except for bare feet or hands), and practitioners use thumb and finger techniques on specific points. Massage sessions usually involve more exposed skin, oils, and longer, sweeping strokes over large areas. If you seek a full-body relaxation effect, massage may be more suitable, while reflexology is ideal for those wanting focused work on specific systems.

How Often Should You Practice Reflexology?

The frequency of reflexology sessions depends on individual needs and wellness goals.

Beginners may benefit from weekly sessions to start, as this frequency helps the body adapt to the therapy and enhances the therapeutic effects.

Weekly appointments can provide stress relief and may even help to address minor, chronic discomforts as the body gradually responds to reflex stimulation.

For those using reflexology for general relaxation and wellness, biweekly or monthly sessions are often enough to maintain a sense of balance and prevent tension build-up. People with specific wellness goals or health concerns might need more frequent sessions, while others might opt for fewer sessions once their issues improve.

Listening to your body is key; if you feel refreshed and balanced, you can adjust the frequency accordingly.

Maintenance sessions every few weeks can support lasting benefits, especially if reflexology is part of a broader wellness routine. Remember, consistency enhances reflexology's effects, so find a rhythm that suits your lifestyle and stick to it for the best results. Communicating with your reflexologist about your wellness goals can also guide the best frequency for you.

How Long Do Reflexology Benefits Last?

The duration of reflexology benefits varies depending on the individual, frequency of sessions, and specific health goals.

For many, relaxation and stress relief are immediate, with effects lasting from a few hours to a few days. Regular sessions can build on these benefits, with many people finding that they feel balanced and relaxed for longer periods as they continue with reflexology.

If reflexology is used to help with chronic issues, such as headaches, insomnia, or digestive problems, benefits may take time to build and may last longer with each session. For example, someone struggling with tension headaches may find relief that initially lasts a few hours but may extend with consistent therapy. Reflexology stimulates the body's healing processes, so lasting benefits depend on how frequently one practices and how the body responds over time.

To maximize and maintain these benefits, incorporating reflexology as part of a broader wellness plan is recommended.

Paired with stress management, balanced nutrition, and regular exercise, reflexology can become a foundational part of a healthy lifestyle, with benefits that compound and sustain over the long term.

When To Avoid Or Limit Reflexology

While reflexology is beneficial for many, there are situations where it's best to avoid or limit this therapy.

Individuals with severe foot injuries, infections, or open wounds should wait until fully healed before trying reflexology, as it could aggravate the injury. Additionally, people with blood clotting disorders or active thrombosis should consult a doctor, as even light pressure could affect circulation.

Pregnant women should approach reflexology with caution, especially in the first trimester. Certain reflex points are thought to stimulate reproductive organs, so it's wise to work with a reflexologist who is experienced in prenatal reflexology if choosing this therapy during pregnancy. People with heart issues, diabetes, or neurological disorders should also discuss their conditions with a healthcare provider to determine if reflexology is appropriate.

If you are undergoing treatment for a serious illness or recovering from surgery, it may be best to wait until your condition stabilizes. Reflexology aims to complement wellness, so if any health issue could be impacted by this therapy, it's essential to get a medical opinion first.

Practicing caution ensures that reflexology remains a safe, enjoyable experience that supports overall wellness.

CHAPTER TEN

Reflexology FAQs And Troubleshooting

When starting with reflexology, common questions often arise about what to expect and how to handle challenges. For beginners, it's essential to understand that each body is unique, and experiences may vary. Reflexology works by applying pressure to reflex points in the feet, hands, or ears, corresponding to specific organs and systems in the body. If you're not seeing immediate results, patience is key. The body might need a few sessions to respond to the therapy.

If you encounter challenges such as missing reflex points or uneven pressure, troubleshooting can help.

Ensure you're using the right amount of pressure—too much or too little can affect the session's effectiveness. It's also helpful to keep detailed notes after each session, tracking how the body reacts. This practice helps in identifying areas that might need more attention or different pressure techniques.

In terms of discomfort, it's common to experience slight tenderness on specific points. However, severe pain indicates that you may be applying too much pressure or that the client is too sensitive in that area. Always communicate with the client and adjust the pressure as needed to ensure a comfortable experience.

How To Handle Sensitive Reflex Points

Sensitive reflex points are areas on the feet or hands that may feel tender when pressure is applied. These points could indicate an imbalance or issue within the corresponding body system. To handle this, it's important to apply pressure gently at first and gauge the person's reaction. You can then gradually increase the pressure, allowing the body to adjust to the sensation.

One effective technique is to use a rotating thumb or finger movement over the sensitive area. This action allows the pressure to remain constant but spread out, minimizing discomfort. If the sensitivity persists, you can alternate between pressing and releasing the point, giving the body time to absorb the stimulation.

Communication with the client is crucial when dealing with sensitive reflex points. Always ask how they feel during the session. If any area is too painful, reduce the pressure immediately. Over time, consistent but gentle work on sensitive points can help reduce tenderness and improve overall balance in the body.

What If You Can't Feel Reflex Points?

For beginners, finding reflex points might be a bit challenging at first. Reflex points can feel like small, raised areas or slightly tender spots under your fingers. If you're struggling to find them, start by using a reflexology chart to guide you. This visual reference will help you locate the general area of each reflex point on the feet or hands.

If you still can't feel them, try adjusting the pressure. Apply firm but controlled pressure with your thumb or fingers. Move slowly across the areas where the reflex points should be, and focus on any subtle changes in texture, firmness, or sensation. You might also feel a small knot or a slight resistance, which could indicate a reflex point.

Keep in mind that practice makes perfect. Over time, your ability to recognize reflex points will improve. It's also helpful to get feedback from the person you're working on. They might feel a sensation even if you're unsure of the point, which can guide you toward better accuracy.

Addressing Soreness After A Session

Soreness after a reflexology session can occur, especially for first-timers or if certain reflex points are particularly sensitive. This reaction is generally a normal part of the body's healing process, indicating that energy is moving through the body's systems. To address this, advise the client to rest and drink plenty of water after the session to help flush out toxins that may have been released during the treatment.

Applying a warm compress to sore areas can also help relieve discomfort. Gentle stretching of the feet or hands and light massage can loosen up tight muscles and reduce soreness. Encourage clients to relax, as stress can intensify post-session tenderness.

If the soreness persists for more than 48 hours, it might indicate that the pressure applied during the session was too intense. In future sessions, use lighter pressure, especially on sensitive areas. Always check in with the client about how they feel throughout the treatment to prevent any excessive discomfort.

How To Improve Your Reflexology Technique

Improving your reflexology technique requires consistent practice and attention to detail. One of the best ways to refine your skills is to maintain a soft yet firm pressure, ensuring the person you're working with is comfortable while still stimulating the reflex points. It's crucial to practice the thumb-walking technique, a foundational skill where you apply pressure by bending and unbending the thumb as you move along the reflex zones.

Another tip for improving your technique is to focus on feedback. Always ask the person about their comfort level and adjust the pressure accordingly. Each client may have different sensitivity levels, so adaptability is key. Use relaxation techniques like slow, rhythmic movements to ease tension before working on more sensitive reflex points.

Finally, continue learning by attending workshops or watching instructional videos to observe how professionals apply pressure and handle different situations. Reflexology is a skill that improves with experience, and being open to new techniques will make you more effective in delivering relief and balance to those you work on.

FAQs On Reflexology Myths And Misconceptions

There are many myths surrounding reflexology, one of the most common being that it's a cure-all treatment. Reflexology is not a cure but rather a complementary therapy that supports the body's natural healing processes. It works best when combined with a healthy lifestyle, proper nutrition, and other medical treatments if needed.

Another misconception is that reflexology is painful. While some reflex points may be tender due to imbalances, the practice should not cause significant pain. Skilled reflexologists use gentle techniques that adjust to the comfort level of the individual, ensuring a soothing experience.

Lastly, some people believe that reflexology only works on the feet. While foot reflexology is common, reflex points are also found on the hands, ears, and even the face. These different areas can be used to target specific body systems, making reflexology a versatile therapy for overall wellness.

Conclusion

The conclusion of a Complete Guide to Reflexology highlights the significant potential of reflexology as a holistic health practice. Reflexology, rooted in ancient healing traditions, emphasizes the connection between various reflex points on the feet, hands, and ears with specific organs, glands, and systems in the body. By applying pressure to these reflex points, practitioners believe that reflexology stimulates the body's natural healing processes, promotes relaxation, and balances physical and emotional well-being.

A comprehensive guide to reflexology also underscores the importance of understanding the anatomy and physiology behind each reflex point. This knowledge empowers practitioners to deliver effective and targeted treatments for common issues such as stress, headaches, digestion, and chronic pain.

Furthermore, this guide typically encourages self-care and at-home practices, which allow individuals to benefit from reflexology between professional sessions. This empowers readers to incorporate reflexology into their routines, either as a standalone practice or in conjunction with other therapeutic approaches.

The guide emphasizes that, while reflexology can be an effective complementary therapy, it should not replace medical care for serious conditions. Reflexology works best when used alongside conventional medicine as a complementary therapy, helping to manage symptoms and improve overall well-being. Thus, a well-rounded understanding of reflexology involves recognizing its boundaries, focusing on holistic support, and aligning with medical advice when necessary.

In summary, a Complete Guide to Reflexology offers readers a thorough understanding of this healing practice, enabling them to harness reflexology's benefits responsibly. With a focus on whole-body wellness, stress relief, and natural healing, the guide serves as both an educational resource and a practical tool, encouraging readers to embrace reflexology as a valuable addition to their self-care and wellness routines.

THE END